ELHEM JBEBLI
SAMAR RHAYEM

Food beliefs in pediatric oncology

ELHEM JBEBLI
SAMAR RHAYEM

Food beliefs in pediatric oncology

True from false

ScienciaScripts

Imprint

Cover image: www.ingimage.com

This book is a translation from the original published under ISBN 978-620-6-71784-3.

Publisher:
Sciencia Scripts
is a trademark of
Dodo Books Indian Ocean Ltd. and OmniScriptum S.R.L publishing group

120 High Road, East Finchley, London, N2 9ED, United Kingdom
Str. Armeneasca 28/1, office 1, Chisinau MD-2012, Republic of Moldova, Europe
Printed at: see last page
ISBN: 978-620-7-91251-3

TABLE OF CONTENTS

INTRODUCTION

Over the last 50 years, the role of diet as a potentially modifiable risk factor in the development of disease has grown steadily [1]. Since the early 1970s, numerous fundamental, clinical and epidemiological research studies have sought to identify and clarify the role of certain nutritional factors likely to act as risk or protective factors in the development of cancers. Since the 1990s, several landmark collective expert reports on nutrition and adult cancer have assessed the results of this work. They have identified relationships between nutrition and adult cancer with varying degrees of certainty [2]. Indeed, some studies estimate that 35% of all cancer deaths are potentially preventable by a change in diet, with a range from 10 to 70% [3].

In the case of children with cancer, nutrition is also part of an overall patient management strategy. Nutritional interventions can benefit cancer survivors by improving quality of life and reducing tumour recurrence. However, given the complexity of research in this field, the evidence is too limited to allow specific recommendations to be drawn up [4].

In the absence of clear recommendations, we are faced with a number of questions about the quality of the education received by mothers of children with cancer regarding their children's diet during and after treatment, and its impact on daily practices in relation to this health problem. The literature searches we carried out did not provide any answers to our questions, as there are very few studies on this subject.

To complete our studies in paediatric care, we are proposing to carry out a project on nutrition in children with cancer through a cross-sectional study of knowledge, attitudes and practices in the oncology unit of the Béchir Hamza Children's Hospital in Tunis. Our objectives are t:

1. To analyse the knowledge, attitudes and practices of mothers in this unit with regard to feeding children with cancer.

2. To identify the factors influencing mothers' knowledge, attitudes and practices with regard to feeding children with cancer

METHODS

1. Type of survey :

This is an observational, cross-sectional, single-centre study. It is descriptive, detailing the knowledge, attitudes and practices of mothers with regard to the diet of their children with cancer.

2. Scope of the survey :

This study was carried out in the oncology unit of the children's medicine department A of the Béchir Hamza children's hospital in Tunis. This unit was chosen in order to recruit a representative sample of the target population, since it collects the majority of children under 15 years of age in the north of Tunisia who are being followed up for a solid tumour.

3. Duration of the survey :

The survey took place over a period of 14 days from 04/02/2019 to 17/02/2019.

4. Study population :

This is a group of mothers recruited from the unit in question.

✓ **Inclusion criteria :**

- All mothers of children being monitored for tumour pathology and treated with chemotherapy.

- Having attended a discussion with one of the doctors in charge of this unit about their children's diet at the time of diagnosis and before the start of treatment; in fact, this discussion is systematically held by the doctors treating all mothers of children with cancer who are about to start chemotherapy treatment.

- Who agreed to answer our questionnaire.

✓ **Non-inclusion criteria :**

- Mothers whose child has already been treated for another tumour pathology or who have another family member who has been treated with chemotherapy. This group of mothers have some prior knowledge of the subject studied.

- Mothers of children with cancer who have another chronic illness. The latter alone may be responsible for the change in eating behaviour.
- The mothers of children whose progress was rapidly fatal. In this situation, the mothers are in a state of stress that prevents them from answering the questionnaire properly.

✓ **Exclusion criteria :**

- Mothers who did not want to answer all the questions, making their questionnaires unusable.

5. **Data collection tools :**

We carried out a knowledge, attitudes and practices survey using a questionnaire comprising 3 main parts: (Appendix I) :
❖ First part: Identification of the children followed: age, diagnosis, length of follow-up, diet. And identification of the mothers: level of education and socio-economic status.
❖ Second part: assessment of mothers' theoretical knowledge about feeding a child with cancer,
❖ Part 3: Assessment of mothers' attitudes and practices regarding the diet of their children undergoing cancer treatment.

The questions were translated into Tunisian dialect. The terms used were defined before the survey began.

6. Data entry and analysis :

The data were analysed manually and then entered using the "Statistical Package for Social Sciences" SPSS version 20 for Windows. The results were represented graphically using EXCEL 2016. Frequencies were compared using the chi-square test or Fischer's exact test, and means were compared using Student's t test. Correlations between the different parameters were assessed using the Pearson correlation test. Differences were considered significant when p was less than 0.05.

7. Bibliographic research :

Bibliographic searches using different keywords relating to the theme under study were carried out on the following sites:

www.pubmed.com www.sciencedirecte.com www.googlescholar.com

8. Ethical considerations :

Before starting data collection, authorisation was obtained from the doctors in charge of the unit concerned. The objectives and procedures of the study were clearly explained to the mothers approached so that they could give free and informed consent. Participation in the study was voluntary with oral consent. All eligible mothers were free to accept or refuse to participate in the study. Anonymity will be respected at all stages of the study.

RESULTS

3.1 Response rate :

46 eligible mothers were approached during the survey, only one of whom refused to answer the questionnaire (response rate = 98%). All completed questionnaires were analysed (N=45).

3.2. Socio-demographic characteristics of the study population:

3.2.1. Age distribution of mothers :

The average age of the mothers was 35 ± 1 year, with extremes ranging from 26 to 35 years. The age distribution of the mothers is shown in Figure 1 [Fig 1], with more than two-thirds of the mothers in their fourth decade.

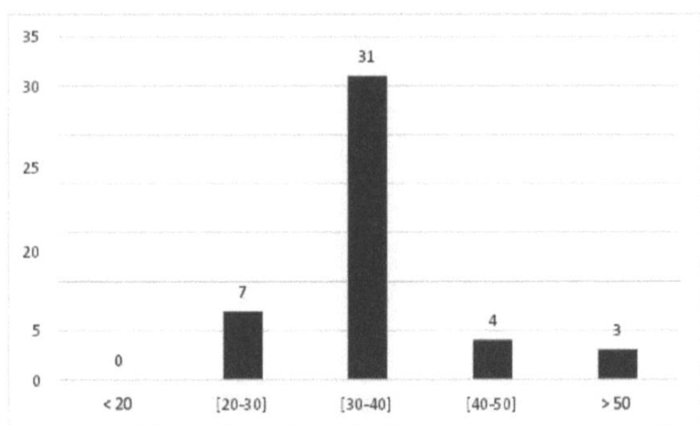

Figure 1: Breakdown of mothers by age

3.2.2. Breakdown by age of child :

The average age of the children was 4 ± 0.42 years, ranging from three months to 14 years. 93.3% of the children were over the age of diversification and 8% were at puberty [Fig 2]. The latter are more difficult to convince to accept a change in their diet.

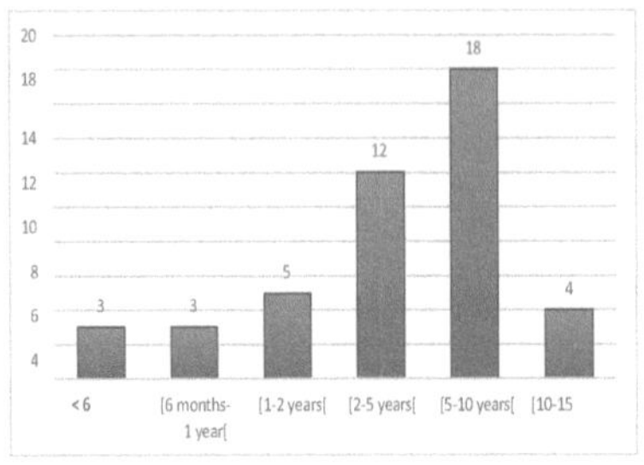

Figure 2: Distribution of patients according to age.

3.2.3. Breakdown by level of education :

The average level of education was 10 years ± 0.86 years, with extremes ranging from 0 (illiterate) to 18 years (Master's degree) [Fig 3]. 64% of the mothers had a good level of education, giving them a good understanding of the importance of diet as a pillar of the multidisciplinary management of children with cancer, and better adherence to the advice given by doctors.

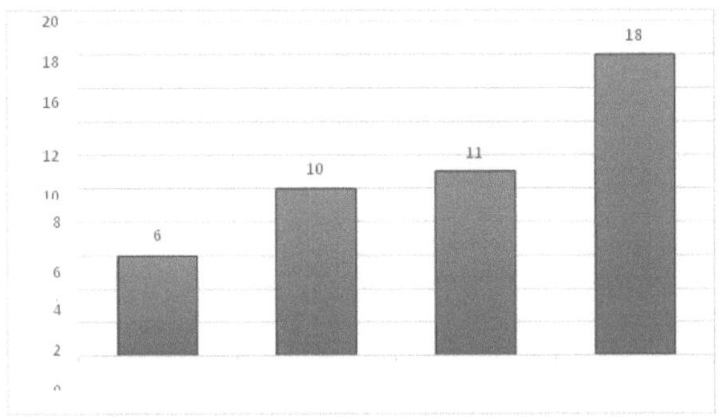

Figure 3: Distribution of mothers by level of education.

3.2.4. Breakdown by positive diagnosis :

The majority of patients were being followed for tumours treated by cures which require the hospitalisation of the child accompanied by his mother every three weeks (74%), i.e. patients being followed for a neuroblastoma, a germ cell tumour, a rhabdomyosarcoma or a lymphoma. Between treatments, however, all the children were seen in day hospital for twice-weekly check-ups [Fig 4]. This hospital presence facilitates access to information provided by health professionals.

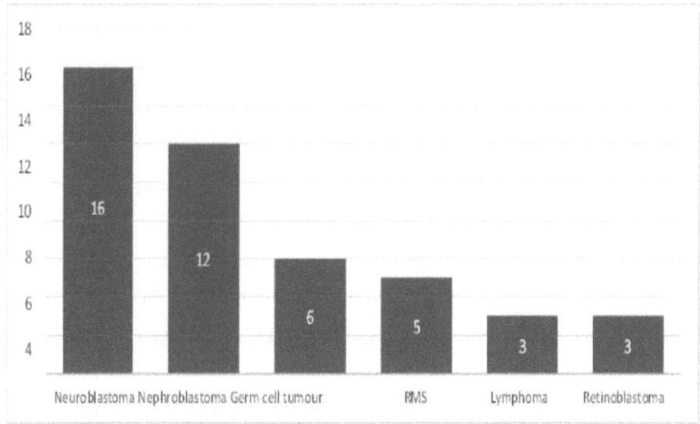

Figure 4:Breakdown of children by pathology.

3.2.5. Breakdown by length of follow-up :

The average follow-up time for our patients was 19 months, with extremes ranging from three months to 32 months [Fig 5].

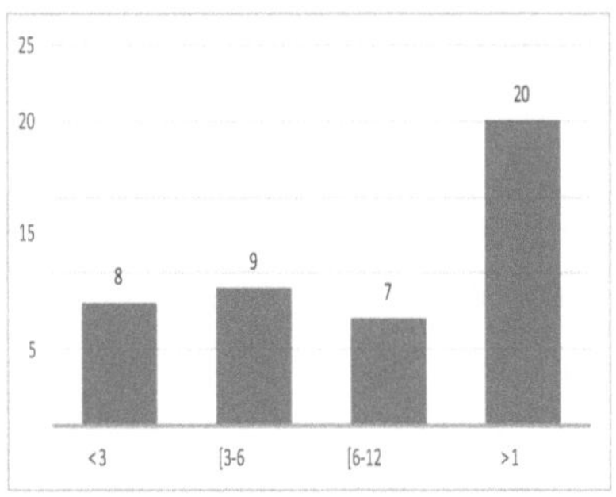

Figure 5: Distribution of children according to length of follow-up.

3.2.6. Distribution according to diet quality prior to diagnosis :

We detailed the children's diet before the positive diagnosis of the tumour to assess the quality of this diet:

Breastfeeding:

The average duration of breastfeeding was 13 months, with extremes ranging from zero to 36 months.

Age of diversification :

The average age of diversification was six months, with extremes ranging from three months to 12 months [Fig 6].

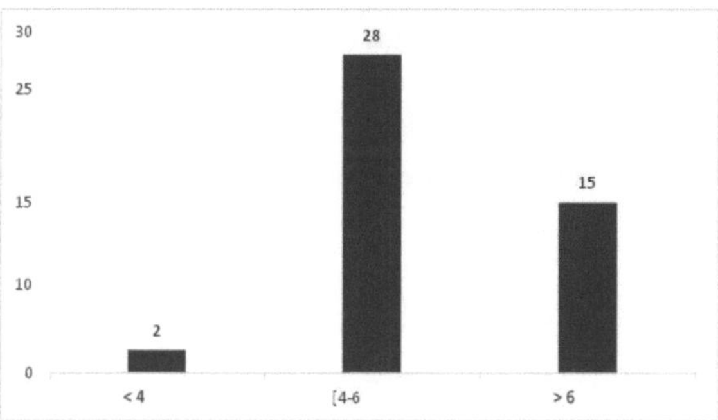

Figure 6: Distribution of children according to age at dietary diversification.

Pace of diversification :

The order in which the different foods were introduced and the time between introductions were respected by 27 children (64.3%).

3.3. Assessment of mothers' knowledge about feeding a child with cancer :

3.3.1. Initial maintenance :

100% of mothers said that they had had an initial meeting with their children's GPs to hear about the disease and to explain how their children would be cared for.

3.3.2. Power supply maintenance :

Only 57.8% of the mothers recalled that the treating doctors had talked about their children's diet during the treatment at the initial interview.

3.3.3. Advice given during the interview:

We asked, without giving any suggestions, what advice had been given during this interview. The spontaneous responses were as follows [Fig 7]:

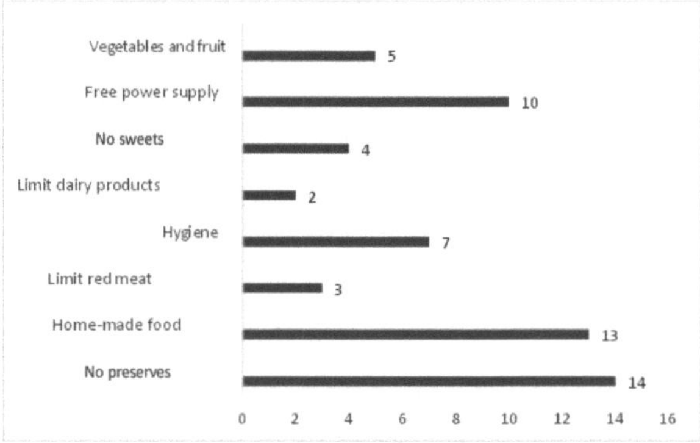

Figure 7: Advice given by mothers during the initial interview.

3.3.4. The importance of diet in the management of children with cancer :

Two-thirds of mothers (29/45) thought that diet played a very important role in the management of their children's illness. Only 8% of mothers said that diet was not important in managing their children's illness [Fig 8].

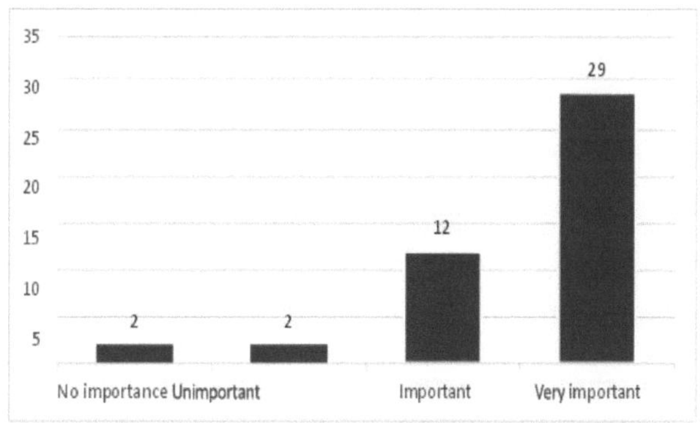

Figure 8:The important role of nutrition in the management of a child with cancer.

3.3.5. Existence of foods with a curative role :

A third of the mothers thought that there was a food whose regular consumption could help their children recover. The remaining mothers were divided between those who did not think such an effect existed (42.2%) and those who did not know (26.7%) [Fig 9].

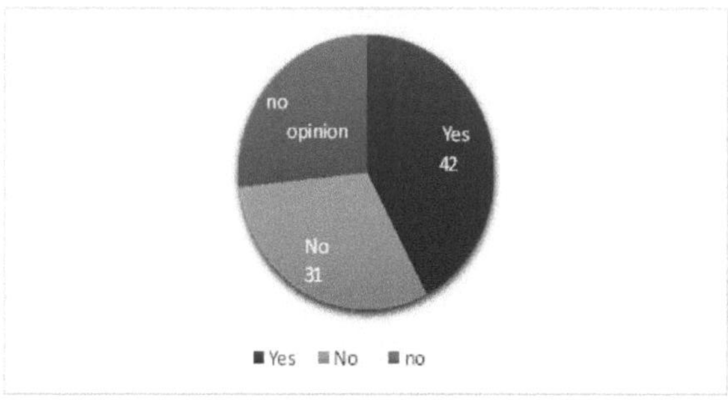

Figure 9:Opinion on the existence of a food with a curative role.

3.3.6. Foodstuffs that accelerate recovery from aplasia :

95.6% of mothers believed in the existence of a food that could accelerate the recovery from aplasia. The foods cited are shown in the following figure [Fig 10]. The foods most frequently mentioned were fruit, dried fruit and vegetables.

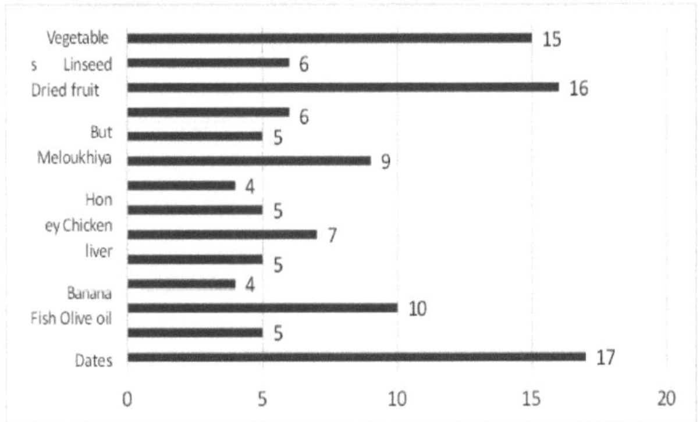

Figure10: Opinion on the existence of a food that stimulates immunity.

3.3.7. Mothers' knowledge of each type of food: We asked mothers to specify which of the foods eaten by their children they thought were beneficial to their children's health. All the mothers thought that vegetables and fruit had a beneficial effect. Two-thirds felt the same way about meat, cereals and dairy products [Fig 11].

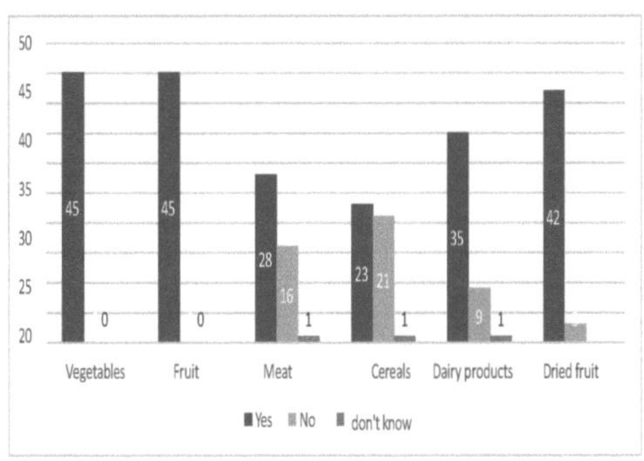

Figure11: Mothers' knowledge of each type of feed.

We named certain foods to the mothers and asked them if they were important for their children's nutrition. The results are shown in Figure 12, which shows that the majority of mothers said so for dried fruit, honey, milk and wholemeal bread [Fig 12].

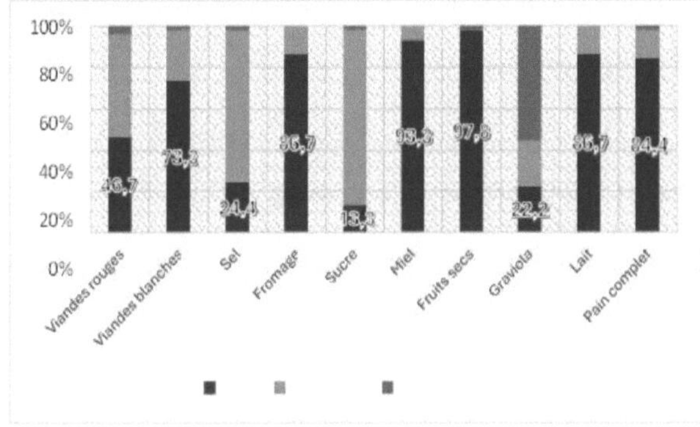

Figure 12: Importance of food according to mothers.

When asked to rank them in descending order of importance, 95.6% of mums thought that vegetables and fruit were the most important, followed by dried fruit (15.4%).

3.3.8. Mothers' knowledge of types of meat: 92% of mothers thought that fish was the most beneficial type of meat, as opposed to white meat (9%) and red meat (0%) [Fig 13].

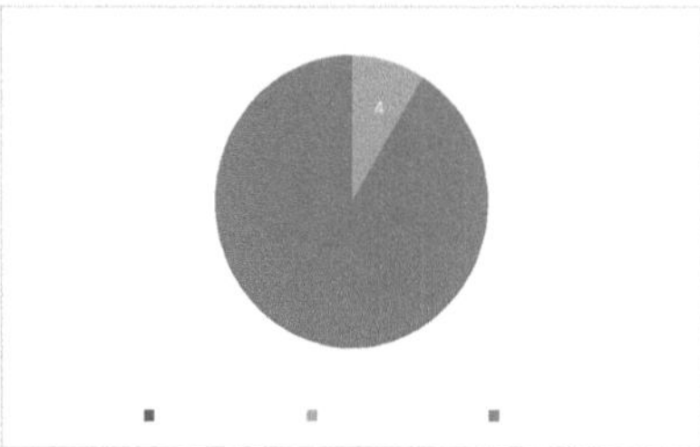

Figure 13: Mothers' knowledge of meat types.

3.4. Evaluation of mothers' feeding practices for a child with cancer:

3.4.1. Regarding the application of the advice given by doctors: 62.2% of mothers said that they had applied the advice given by their GPs during the initial interview.

3.4.2. Changes in their children's eating habits :

49% of mothers said they had changed their eating habits since their children were diagnosed with the disease.

3.4.3. Type of change in eating habits :

Changes in eating habits included a reduction in the consumption of tinned food in 20% of cases, red meat in 11.1% of cases and fried food in 5% of cases. On the other hand, there was an increase in the consumption of vegetables and fruit in 22.2% of cases, fish in 9% of cases and turmeric in 4.4% of cases.

3.4.4. Aspects of changes in eating habits :

84.4% of mothers said that they placed the greatest emphasis on the hygiene of the food, 4.4% placed the greatest emphasis on quality, while 2.2% placed the greatest emphasis on the quantity of food ingested [Fig 14].

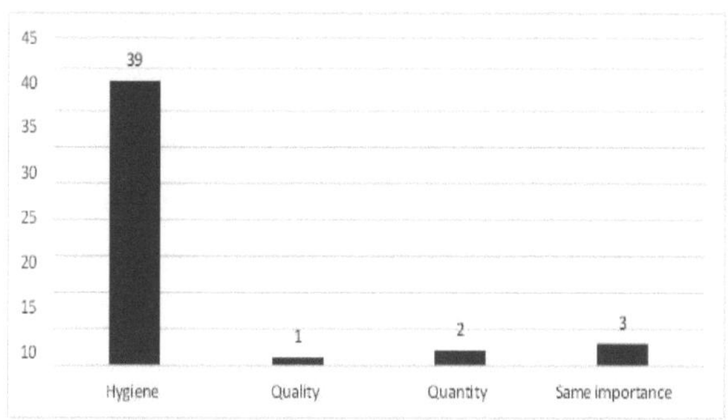

Figure 14: Aspects of changes in eating behaviour.

When the mothers were asked to rank these aspects of eating behaviour in order of importance, the results showed that hygiene came first. (91% of cases), quality came second (62% of cases) and quantity third (65% of cases) [Fig 15].

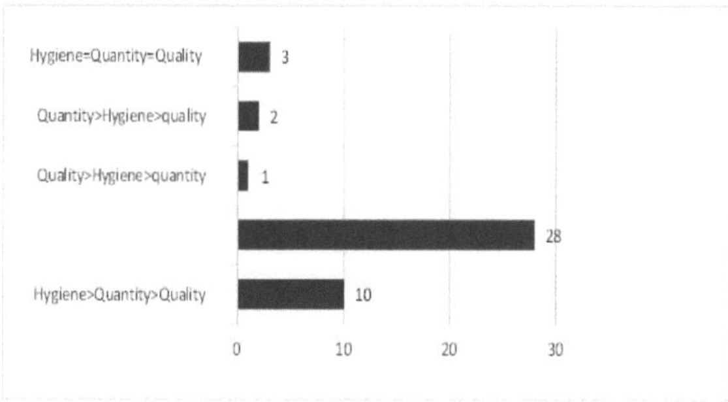

Figure 15: Order of importance of the different aspects of diet.

3.4.5. Reasons for changes in eating habits :

The first reason for modifying the dietary habits of children with cancer was to stimulate the immune system in order to speed up recovery from aplasia in 60% of patients. Chemotherapy-induced aplasia is not only a condition that favours the onset of sometimes serious infections, but also the main cause of delays in chemotherapy treatments, as this delay in treatment planning is itself a factor in poor prognosis for tumour pathologies. The second cause was accelerated healing in 45% of cases. The other causes are summarised in Figure 16 [Fig 16].

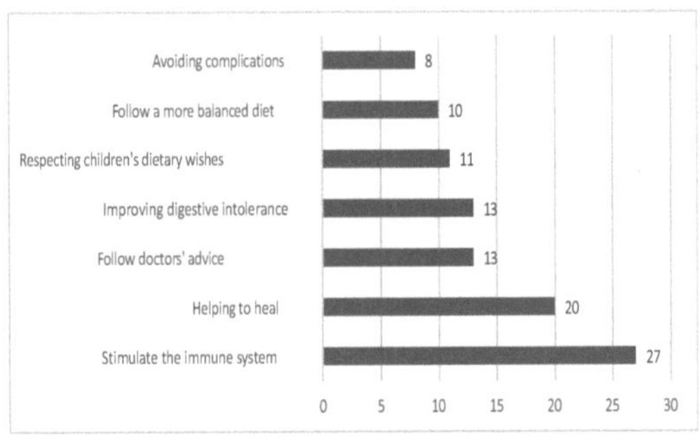

Figure 16: Causses of changes in eating habits.

3.4.6. Use of food supplements :

26% of mothers said that they had given their children food supplements at the same time as the chemotherapy treatment. These supplements were vitamins (10 cases), proteins and amino acids (three cases) and trace elements (one case). The use of these food supplements was prescribed by a doctor in four cases, at the suggestion of family and friends in two cases, and on the mothers' own initiative in six cases.

3.4.7. Sources of information about feeding children with cancer:

The primary source of information about the diet of children with cancer was the doctors treating them in 78% of cases. However, the mothers also referred to other non-professional sources of information, such as the mothers of other children being treated in the same oncology unit, family and friends, or electronic sources and social networks in almost a third of cases each [Fig17].

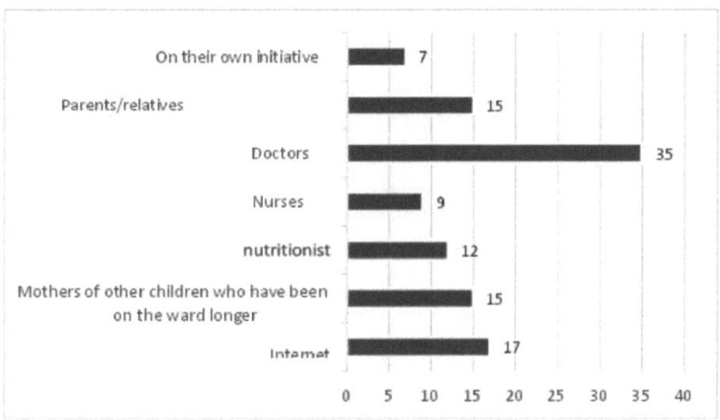

Figure 17: Mums' sources of information about the diet of their children with cancer.

3.4.8. Source of children's food :

69% of mothers said that they only gave their children homemade food, while 31% gave them purchased food in one-third of cases and unpackaged food handled with the hands in one-third of cases [Fig 18].

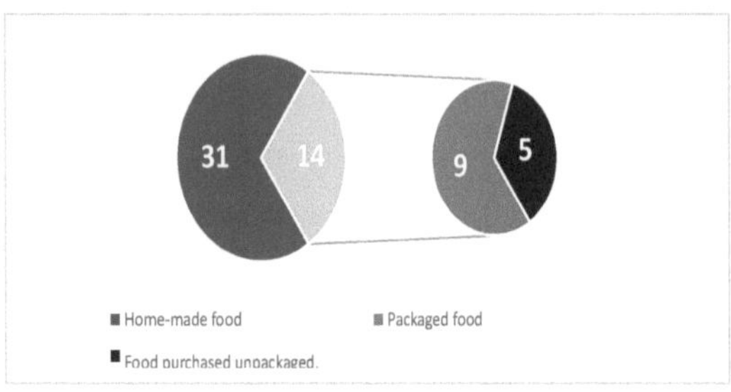

Figure18: The source of food consumed.

3.5. Research into factors associated with mothers' knowledge, attitudes and practices regarding the diet of their children with cancer:

In analysing our results, we carried out a uni-variate study to look for factors associated with mothers' knowledge or attitudes and practices. Some factors were identified. After analysing the data collection forms one by one, our study population was divided into two groups: the first was made up of mothers whose knowledge and practices regarding their children's diet were correct (n=28) and the second was made up of mothers whose knowledge and practices were judged to be incorrect (n=17). The factors studied were: mother's age, child's age, positive diagnosis, length of follow-up in the oncology unit, mother's level of education, socio-economic level and initial interview about feeding. The results show that :

- The mothers' age, the child's age, the positive diagnosis, the length of follow-up and the initial interview about feeding were not factors that had a significant impact on the mothers' knowledge and practices.
- Mums' knowledge and practices regarding the diet of children with cancer were significantly influenced by :

- Family socio-economic level ($p = 0.003$).
- Mother's level of education ($p = 0.002$).

DISCUSSION

This study looked at the dietary beliefs of mothers of children with cancer through a descriptive and analytical cross-sectional study conducted at the Paediatric Oncology Unit of the Béchir Hamza Children's Hospital in Tunis, which yielded 45 observations.The response rate in our series was 97.8%, which is a high rate, reflecting the interest in the subject shown by the mothers we spoke to. Studies have shown that 15% to 40% of cancer patients lose weight during treatment. This percentage can rise to 85% in patients with advanced disease [5]. Consequently, early intervention and education of patients about their nutrition and eating habits can improve these results and prevent such complications. Improved nutritional support leads to reduced morbidity and mortality, shorter hospital stays and lower management costs [6,7].

In our study, all the mothers stated that they had had an initial interview with the doctors treating them to announce the disease and to explain how their children would be cared for. Only 57.8% said that the doctors had discussed their children's diet during treatment at this meeting. Nutritional assessment is an important element in the management of tumour pathologies. It is defined as the advice and education given to change patients' eating habits and behaviour. It is extremely important to provide optimal care to minimise the complications associated with weight loss and undernutrition [8].

A growing body of evidence suggests that diet and body weight can influence the health of cancer survivors [9]. Due to the complexity of this area of research, the evidence is too limited to develop specific recommendations. Therefore, current recommendations for cancer survivors are based more on primary prevention recommendations [4].

As both a risk factor and a protective factor, nutrition is one of the behavioural factors that can be influenced as part of the fight against cardiovascular disease. cancer prevention [10]. Furthermore, the results of randomised controlled trials on diet and prognosis are limited and show mixed results [11].

4.1. Recommendations concerning the diet of children with cancer:

The guidelines recommend that macro- and micronutrient intakes should be adequate during treatment, while any form of diet not based on clinical evidence is strongly discouraged. In addition, current dietary advice for cancer patients consists of personalised advice from a qualified professional, based on site, nutritional status and treatment toxicity [4,12]. Other studies indicate that Western-type dietary profiles are associated with an increased risk of several cancers and, conversely, 'health-promoting' dietary profiles are associated with a decreased risk of prevalence of several cancers. However, significant heterogeneity has been observed between the studies included in the meta-analyses; this can be explained in part by differences in the share attributed to each of the factors used to construct the dietary profiles and scores [10]. The protective or favourable role of the various nutrients in paediatric cancers is unclear, as very few studies have looked into this subject, unlike in adults, where the causal link or protective role of certain foods has been well described, with varying levels of evidence [Appendix 2].

With regard to types of meat, 92% of the mothers questioned thought that fish was the most beneficial type of meat, as opposed to white meat (9%) and red meat (0%). A recent systematic review, including different types of cancer, indicates that high intakes of fish are inversely associated with overall mortality [13].

In this study, all the mothers thought that vegetables and fruit had a beneficial effect on their children's health. The meta-analyses show a significant reduction in the risk of cancer of the mouth, pharynx and larynx of 28% with vegetables (non-starchy), 29% with raw vegetables and 24% with citrus fruit, for an increase in intake of 50g/day, and 28% with fruit. fruit for an increase in intake of 100 g/day [10]. They confirmed a reduction in the risk of oesophageal cancer and colorectal cancer with a "suggested" level of evidence associated with fibre consumption [10]. Conversely, in another study, consumption of more than five portions of fruit and vegetables a day, high fibre intake and low fat intake did not affect prognosis [14].

One third of the mothers included in this study thought that red meat was not beneficial in this context. In the literature, the data published on the association between digestive cancers and meat consumption allow us to retain this significant association with a "convincing" level of evidence [10].

The majority of our patients' mothers had insisted on the beneficial role of dairy products. Experts consider that milk consumption is associated with a reduced risk of colorectal cancer with a "probable" level of evidence, and that cheese consumption is associated with an increased risk with a "suggested" level of evidence [10]. A meta-analysis of nine cohort studies showed a significant reduction (10%) in the risk of colorectal cancer per 200 g/day portion of milk. The results of the dose-response analysis support a non-linear association. The reduction in colorectal cancer risk is small below 200 g/day, but becomes significant (20-30% reduction observed) when milk intake is between 500 and 800 g/day [10]. The proportion attributable to salt consumption is estimated to be 0.9% in men and 0.2% in women for all cancer sites combined, and 24% for stomach cancers [10]. In this study, more than 70% of mothers were aware of the harmful effects of salt consumption on their children.

According to WCRF/AICR estimates, around 1/4 of all cancers (1/3 of the most common cancers) in developed countries and 1/5 in developing countries could be prevented by a change in lifestyle that incorporates nutritional recommendations (a diet rich in fruit and vegetables and fibre, with no excess of red meat, cold meats or salt, regular physical activity and a normal weight) [10]. The weakness of these studies is that they are less informative in terms of prevention than data on incidence, because they are linked to both incidence and incidence rates. early management and treatment options. When each nutritional factor and cancer site is considered, estimates of the proportion attributable to diet range from 2.7% to 65.2%. Given the many methodological limitations of these studies, these estimates should not be considered definitive. They do, however, highlight the potential for prevention associated with these factors, considered separately or as a whole [10].

Considering the diet as a whole, higher dietary quality scores and cautious/healthy diets were associated with a decreased risk of mortality in cancer survivors, while Western diets had the opposite effect [13]. Nutrition following Western diets also showed a higher risk of recurrence and mortality compared to those following a prudent diet, in a prospective study of 1009 colorectal cancer survivors [15].

4.2. Practices relating to food and cancer :

49% of the mothers questioned said that they had changed their eating habits since their children were diagnosed with cancer. In fact, cancer patients tend to change their eating habits once they have been diagnosed with cancer, often turning to the Internet for information on non-specific treatments, which may even be harmful [16]. Changes in diet have been reported in several studies [10,13,14]. A reduction in milk and dairy products was reported in 61% of patients. This change was also observed in a prospective study conducted in France, where data were collected from dietary records and compared before and after cancer diagnosis [14,17,18].A very small percentage of patients reported an increase in fruit and vegetable consumption. This is not in line with the WCRF recommendations. This may be reasonable for patients with gastrointestinal symptoms due to cancer or its treatment, but less understandable for patients wishing to improve their health. However, we do not We cannot exclude the fact that these patients have already eaten the recommended amount of fruit and vegetables. A prospective study conducted in France [14] reported a reduction in vegetable consumption, while an increase in fruit consumption was observed in the same population. In the UK, an increase in the number of fruit and vegetables eaten was also observed using a semi-quantitative meal frequency questionnaire to compare dietary changes before and after diagnosis [13].

□ **Types of changes in eating habits :**

In this study, changes in eating habits involved a reduction in the consumption of tinned food in 20% of cases, red meat in 11.1% of cases and fried food in 5% of cases. On the other hand, an increase in the consumption of vegetables and fruit was observed in 22.2% of cases, fish in 9% of cases and turmeric in 4.4% of cases. Many cancer patients make positive, healthy food choices after being diagnosed with cancer. In fact, the majority of studies reviewed reported the adoption of 'healthier diets', including increased consumption of fruit and vegetables, reduced consumption of fat, red meat and sugary foods [19-21]. Healthier food choices have also been observed in other cohorts. For example, in a study of patients who completed a self-administered questionnaire, most survivors reported having reduced their intake of fat, meat, sugar and salt since their diagnosis, eating more fish, vegetables, fruit, fibre, whole grains and water [21].

□ **Causes of changes in eating habits :**

The primary reason for changing the dietary habits of children with cancer was to stimulate the immune system in order to accelerate recovery from chemotherapy-induced aplasia, followed by recovery. The reasons for changing dietary habits have been little reported in the literature. In the work by Salminen et al, the reasons most frequently given were the desire to recover in more than half the patients (52.9%), the relief of certain symptoms such as nausea and to follow the doctor's instructions (11.8% each) [20,22]. In fact, cancer diagnosis and treatment modalities have have serious consequences for patients' nutritional status. They affect the metabolic process and cause loss of appetite. In addition, the use of different cancer treatment modalities, such as chemotherapy, surgery and radiotherapy, leads to numerous side effects, including anorexia, diarrhoea, mouth infections, vomiting, altered taste buds and nausea, all of which affect eating habits and lead to poor nutritional status [23,24]. In another study of Malaysian patients in British Columbia, the most common reason given for changing diet was to follow doctors' instructions (58.2%), while a smaller percentage of patients changed diet because of their increased desire to cure their cancer (35.8%) [25].

□ **Use of food supplements :**

One of the most common changes in the behaviour of cancer patients is the use of dietary supplements. Although many studies on this topic have been carried out in countries where, in the general population, it is very common to use dietary supplements, it has been found that cancer patients are often more likely to use supplements or to start using them after a cancer diagnosis [19- 21,22]. In our study, 26% of mothers had given dietary supplements to their children in parallel with cancer treatment. In the literature, 58% of parents confirmed regular consumption of these supplements. The products most frequently used were vitamins (51%) and aloe vera (29.1%), although there is no evidence that supplements can have an impact on cancer prognosis [26]. Natural" food supplements are frequently used and demanded by cancer patients. As their supposed anti-tumour effects have not yet been demonstrated by appropriate efficacy evaluations, their use cannot be recommended. However, healthcare professionals involved in the nutritional treatment of cancer patients should be informed about this issue so that they can discuss with them the potential risks, benefits and expectations associated with the specific consumption of food supplements. [26]. It also appeared that the use of supplements was more frequent in patients with a higher level of education than those with a lower level, and in younger patients compared with older patients [20,22].

On the other hand, the results of new meta-analyses in adults suggest an increased risk of stomach cancer with the consumption of betacarotene-based dietary supplements with a probable level of evidence [10].

Sources of information about diet Children treated for tumour pathology :

Thanks to advances in new communication technologies, the amount of information available on cancer has exploded [27]. This knowledge is not exclusively available to healthcare professionals, as modern communication channels, such as the internet, are changing the nature and speed of information [28]. The vast amount of readily available information has enormous potential to influence what people know about cancer, but the main challenge lies in the difficulty of separating the quality from the quantity of cancer information.

Our study showed that the primary source of information about the diet of children with cancer was the treating doctor in 78% of cases, but mothers also referred to other non-professional sources of information. A recent study showed that nutritional advice within the hospital was available to only 15% of participants, 26% received general information from an oncologist, while 59% of patients gathered general information from websites, relatives, friends or general nutritionists. In addition, almost all patients (91.2%) expressed the urgent need to receive more information about an appropriate diet directly from the centre where they are treated. These data can be explained by the lack of nutrition awareness among oncologists, the lack of solid evidence of correct diet during treatment and the need for more health professionals trained in nutrition in oncology units [29].As effective communication is considered essential to achieving optimal health outcomes, it is essential that patients understand what and who they need to know about their treatment journey to ensure quality cancer care [30].

4.3. Factors influencing changes in eating habits :

Several factors were studied by univariate analysis, but only two were significantly associated with knowledge and practices concerning the diet of children with cancer: socio-economic level ($p=0.003$) and mother's level of education ($p=0.002$). In fact, these two factors can influence dietary behaviour even in the absence of any tumour pathology. There is almost no data in the literature concerning the significance of these factors.

4.4. Limitations of the study :

Certain biases should be highlighted:

➢ The number of 45 patients may be considered insufficient to assess the knowledge of all mothers of children with cancer in Tunisia. It is true that the Oncology Unit of the Béchir Hamza Children's Hospital in Tunis treats a large number of children with solid tumours, but this unit mainly treats patients from Greater Tunis and the north of Tunisia, which reduces the representativeness of this sample, hence the need to repeat a multicentre study.

➢ The information was collected by means of an interview written in French and the questions were translated into Tunisian dialect at the time of the interview with the mothers. The terms used were defined before the start of the survey. This could introduce bias on the part of the interviewer, despite all the precautions taken. It would be wiser to repeat this study on a larger scale using a questionnaire translated into dialect.

➢ Only qualitative changes and not quantitative aspects of diet were collected.

➢ Eating habits were not assessed and compared before and after diagnosis. The results may be influenced by the general perception of a healthy diet and do not accurately represent changes linked to the nature of the disease.

➢ Few studies have been carried out on the dietary knowledge, attitudes and practices of mothers of children with cancer, which has limited our comments and discussions, sometimes using studies carried out on adults as a reference.

However, despite the limitations of this study, our results offer some insights into the dietary knowledge of children with cancer in Tunisia. Indeed, studies that aim to assess and analyse food-related knowledge, attitudes and practices are a useful method for identifying and exploring the personal factors that determine eating habits. These studies can therefore provide useful information and contribute to the effective planning of programmes and projects. They are also essential when evaluating nutrition communication and education interventions, i.e. activities explicitly aimed at improving people's knowledge, attitudes and practices in relation to nutrition.

4.5. Recommendations:

A number of people are involved in the nutritional management of children with cancer. Paediatric technicians are ideally placed to provide initial assessment and advice [31,32]. However, their ability to provide mothers with nutritional support and advice depends on their knowledge of nutritional assessment and the demands made on them along the way. Alarmingly, in a study by Van Veen et al, 43% of oncology nurses felt that they did not have sufficient knowledge to provide nutritional advice [33].

In order to improve mothers' knowledge and practices, these target mothers need to be offered appropriate health education, from a source capable of providing it. The task is carried out by a team of experts (doctors, nutritionists and paediatricians) at different times:

- Improve awareness and information for mothers about their children's diet (when the diagnosis is announced, during the various courses of chemotherapy, during regular monitoring in the day hospital).
- Correcting false preconceptions, bad habits among mothers concerning their children's nutrition and their behaviour.
- Putting in place educational resources to avoid bad practices on the part of these mothers: providing families with brochures and posters detailing the different aspects of feeding a child with cancer.
- Educational messages must be clear and simplified, easy to assimilate by all mothers, especially those with a low level of education.
- Stress the importance of a balanced diet that respects both the needs of a growing child and the child's illness.
- Provide ongoing training on this subject for nursing staff, particularly those working in paediatric oncology units.

CONCLUSIONS

Nutritional care for children with cancer is one of the pillars of multidisciplinary care. In this study, we set out to evaluate the beliefs, attitudes and practices of mothers concerning the diet of their children undergoing paediatric oncology treatment, in order to determine the factors influencing knowledge and associated with good practice. Our assessment revealed gaps in knowledge at various levels, both theoretical and practical. The factors significantly influencing this knowledge were mothers' level of education and socio-economic status. The level of knowledge and different practices could be improved by awareness-raising campaigns. A national multicentre study is needed to ensure that the results are more representative and can be better interpreted. In this context, the role of paediatricians in the nutritional education of mothers of children with cancer is essential, through education at various stages:

- At the time of diagnosis.
- During hospitalisation.
- At the time of regular check-ups in the day hospital.
- During outpatient follow-up after the end of treatment for cancer survivors.

It is also important to provide parents with documents and aids on the subject of nutrition for children with cancer, detailing the recommendations with a good level of evidence.

REFERENCES

[1] Lim SS, Vos T, Flaxman AD, Danaei G, Shibuya K, Adair-Rohani H, et al. A comparative risk assessment of burden of disease and injury attributable to 67 risk factors and risk factor clusters in 21 regions, 1990-2010: a systematic analysis for the Global Burden of Disease Study 2010. The lancet 2012;380:2224-60.

[2] Ancellin R, Cottet V, D-Pecollo N, L-Martel P, Pierre F, Touillaud M, Touvier M, Vasson M-P. Nutrition et prévention primaire des cancers: actualisation des données, collection État des lieux et des connaissances. Paris: Institut national du cancer; 2015.

[3] Doll R, Peto R. The causes of cancer: quantitative estimates of avoidable risks of cancer in the United States today. J Natl Cancer Inst 1981;66:1191-308.

[4] Rock CL, Doyle C, Demark-Wahnefried W, Meyerhardt J, Courneya KS, Schwartz et al. Nutrition and physical activity guidelines for cancer survivors. CA: a Cancer Journal for Clinicians, 2012;62(4) :243-274.

[5] Omlin A. Nutrition Impact Symptoms In Advanced Cancer Patients: Frequency And Specific Interventions, A Case-Control Study. Journal Of Cachexia, Sarcopenia And Muscle 2013 ;4(1):55-61.

[6]. Fjeldsta, SH. Changes In Nutritional Care After Implementing National Guidelines-A 10-Year Follow-Up Study. European Journal Of Clinical Nutrition,2018:1.

[7]. Kris-Etherton P. The Need To Advance Nutrition Education In The Training Of Health Care Professionals And Recommended Research To Evaluate Implementation And Effectiveness-The American Journal Of Clinical Nutrition. 2014 ;99(5):1153-66.

[8] Hopkinson, J.B., Nutritional Support Of The Elderly Cancer Patient: The Role Of The Nurse. Nutrition. 2015;31(4):598-602.

[9] Pekmezi, D W, Demark-Wahnefried, W. Updated evidence in support of diet and exercise interventions in cancer survivors. Acta Oncologica. 2011;50(2):167-178.

[10] Ancellin R, Cottet V, D-Pecollo N, L-Martel P, Pierre F, Touillaud M et al. Nutrition et prévention primaire des cancers: actualisation des données, collection État des lieux et des connaissances. Paris: Institut national du cancer (INCa); 2015.

[11] Diet, nutrition,physical activity and breast cancer survivors. London :World Cancer Research Fund International, Continuous Update Project;2014.

[12] Arends J, Bachmann P, Baracos V, Barthelemy N, Bertz H, Bozzetti F, et al. ESPEN guidelines on nutrition in cancer patients. Clinical Nutrition 2017;36:11-48.

[13] Schwedhelm C, Boeing H, Hoffmann G, Aleksandrova K, Schwingshackl L. Effect of diet on mortality and cancer recurrence among cancer survivors: a systematic review and meta-analysis of cohort studies. Nutrition reviews 2016;74: 737-748.

[14] Pierce, J. P., Natarajan, L., Caan, B. J., Parker, B. A., Greenberg, E. R., Flatt, S. W et al. Influence of a diet very high in vegetables, fruit, and fiber and low in fat on prognosis following treatment for breast cancer: The Women's Healthy Eating and Living (WHEL) randomized trial. JAMA: The Journal of the American Medical Association. 2017 ;298(3), 289-298.

[15] Meyerhardt, J. A., Niedzwiecki, D., Hollis, D., Saltz, L. B., Hu, F. B., Mayer, R. J., & Fuchs, C. S. (2007). Association of dietary patterns with

cancer recurrence and survival in patients with stage III colon cancer. JAMA: The Journal of the American Medical Association, 298(7), 754-764.

[16] Helft PR, Hlubocky F, Daugherty CK. American Oncologists' Views of Internet Use by Cancer Patients: A Mail Survey of American Society of Clinical Oncology Members. Journal of Clinical Oncology 2003;21:942-7.

[17] Larsson SC, Crippa A, Orsini N, Wolk A, Michaëlsson K. Milk consumption and mortality from all causes, cardiovascular disease, and cancer: a systematic review and meta-analysis. Nutrients 2015; 7(9), 7749-7763.

[18] Pereira PC, Milk nutritional composition and its role in human health. Nutrition 2014; 30(6), 619-627.

[19] Velentzis LS, Keshtgar MR, Woodside JV, Leathem AJ, Titcomb A, Perkins KA, et al. Significant changes in dietary intake and supplement use after breast cancer diagnosis in a UK multicentre study. Breast cancer research and treatment 2011; 128(2), 473-482.

[20] Salminen, E. K., Lagstrom, H. K., Heikkila, S., & Salminen, S. (2000). Does breast cancer change patients' dietary habits? European Journal of Clinical Nutrition, 54(11), 844-848.

[21] Bours, M. J., Beijer, S., Winkels, R. M., van Duijnhoven, F. J., Mols, F., Breedveld- Peters, J. J., & van de Poll-Franse, L. V. (2015). Dietary changes and dietary supplement use, and underlying motives for these habits reported by colorectal cancer survivors of the Patient Reported Outcomes Following Initial Treatment and Long-term Evaluation of Survivorship (PROFILES) registry. The British Journal of Nutrition, 114(2), 286-296.

[22] Salminen, E., Bishop, M., Poussa, T., Drummond, R., & Salminen, S. (2002). Breast cancer patients have unmet needs for dietary advice. Breast, 11(6), 516-521.

[23] Andreoli, A., et al, New Trends In Nutritional Status Assessment Of Cancer Patients. Eur Rev Med Pharmacol Sci, 2011. 15(5): P. 469-480.

[24] Wang, R., Et Al, Impact Exerted By Nutritional Risk Screening On Clinical Outcome Of Patients With Esophageal Cancer. Biomed Research International, 2018:P. 1-5.

[25] Shaharudin, S. H., Sulaiman, S., Shahril, M. R., Emran, N. A., & Akmal, S. N. (2013). Dietary changes among breast cancer patients in Malaysia. Cancer Nursing, 36(2), 131-138.

[26] Frenkel M, Sierpina V. The use of dietary supplements in oncology. Current oncology reports 2014; 16(11), 411.

[27] Viswanath, K., Nagler, R. H., Bigman-Galimore, C. A., McCauley, M. P., Jung, M., & Ramanadhan, S. The communications revolution and health inequalities in the 21st century: Implications for cancer control. Cancer Epidemiology, Biomarkers & Prevention, 2012 October [21/10/2012] ; [24 pages].

[28] Davis, P. M., & Walters, W. H. (2011). The impact of free access to the scientific literature: A review of recent research. Journal of the Medical Library Association, 99(3), 208-217.

[29] Caccialanza R, Cereda E, Pinto C, Cotogni P, Farina G, Gavazzi C, et al. Awareness and consideration of malnutrition among oncologists: insights from an exploratory survey. Nutrition 2016; 32(9), 1028-1032.

[30] Rutten, L. J., Arora, N. K., Bakos, A. D., Aziz, N., & Rowland, J. (2005). Information needs and sources of information among cancer patients: A systematic review of research (1980-2003). Patient Education

and Counseling, 57(3), 250-261.

[31]. Bozzetti, F., et al, The Nutritional Risk In Oncology: A Study Of 1,453 Cancer Outpatients. Supportive Care In Cancer, 2012. 20(8): P. 1919-1928.

[32] Tappenden, K.A., Et Al, Critical Role Of Nutrition In Improving Quality Of Care: An Interdisciplinary Call To Action To Address Adult Hospital Malnutrition. Journal Of Parenteral And Enteral Nutrition, 2013. 37(4): P. 482-497

[33] Van Veen, M.R., Et Al. Improving Oncology Nurses' Knowledge About Nutrition And Physical Activity For Cancer Survivors. In Oncology Nursing Forum; 2017.

APPENDICES

Appendix 1: Data collection form.

A survey of food beliefs mothers of children undergoing paediatric oncology treatment:

File no. :

Date of admission :

Full name :

Date of birth :

Age :

Gender :

Diagnosis :

Mother's level of education: Socio-economic level

Length of follow-up since diagnosis: Weight on admission:

Initial diet:

Breast milk:

Formula milk:

Cow's milk

Age of diversification :

- Vegetables :
- Fruit :
- Cereals :
- Family dish :

Did you have an interview with the doctors when the diagnosis was announced: yes / no.

During this interview, did he talk to you about your child's diet: yes / no.

Which are the advice you a you:

Did you apply the advice given: yes / no

In your opinion, how important is the role of nutrition in the management of a child with cancer?

- very important
- important
- not important
- of any importance.

In your opinion, are there any foods that can help heal your child?

yes / no.

Which ones:

Have you given your child this type of food: yes / no.

Do you continue to give it to her to this day: yes / no

Do you think the following foods are important for your child at the moment?

- Vegetables: yes / no
- Fruit: yes / no
- Meat: yes / no
- Cereals: yes / no
- Milk and dairy products: yes / no
- Others:

Order of importance

descending:

Which of the following is important for meat?

- Red meat
- White meat
- Fish

Order of importance

decreasing

Are there foods that stimulate immunity (what food do you give your child to stimulate immunity): yes / no

Which ones

Have you really changed your child's eating habits: yes / no

What changes :

You place more emphasis on :

- Hygiene
- The quantity
- Quality

The reasons for these changes :

- A more balanced diet
- Helping to heal
- Avoiding complications
- Boosting immunity
- Follow the diet accepted by the child
- Regimen dictated by the location of the tumour
- Reduce digestive symptoms
- Follow doctors' advice

Have you given your child any food supplements: yes

/ no

What type of supplements:

- vitamins
- trace elements
- Protein / AA

Who indicated that these supplements were taken:

- On your own initiative
- Suggestions from friends and family
- The dietician
- Medical indication

When you need information or advice about your child's diet, the source of your information is :

- Mothers of other children who have been on the ward longer
- Internet
- Nutritionist
- Nurses
- The doctors
- Relatives / friends

Assessment of your child's weight since the start of treatment:

- Stable
- Loss
- Gain
- Weight loss then weight gain

According to the mother:initial weight:current weight:

According to the file:initial weight:current weight:

Are these foods good or bad?

- Red meat :
- White meat :
- Salt :
- Cheese :
- Sugar :

- Honey :
- Dried fruit :
- Graviola
- Milk :
- Wholemeal bread

Your child's food source :

- Only home-made food
- Only purchased food
- The two
- If food purchased :packagedunpackaged

Appendix 2: The role of each type of food in preventing or promoting the onset of cancer in adults :

NIVEAUX DE PREUVE DES RELATIONS ENTRE LES FACTEURS NUTRITIONNELS PRÉSENTÉS DANS CE RAPPORT ET DIFFÉRENTES LOCALISATIONS DE CANCERS

	Tumeurs solides																								Hémopathies malignes			
	Nasopharynx	Tête et cou	Bouche (cavité orale), pharynx, larynx	Œsophage	Adénocarcinomes œsogastrique	Estomac	Intestin grêle	Côlon-rectum	Pancréas	Ampoule de Vater	Foie	Vésicule biliaire	Rein	Vessie	Sein (avant la ménopause)	Sein (après la ménopause)	Endomètre	Col de l'utérus	Ovaire	Prostate	Testicule	Poumon	Thyroïde	Peau	Lymphome hodgkinien	Lymphome non hodgkinien	Leucémie	Myélome multiple
Boissons alcoolisées							*	Homme / Femme		*			**										*		*	*		
Surcharge pondérale						* Proximal / Distal					**									** Avancé / Localisé	*	**	*		*	*	*	*
Viandes rouges				**									*	*	*					*								
Charcuteries				**									*	*	*					**		**						
Sel et aliments salés																												
Compléments alimentaire à base de bêtacarotène		*	*	*		* **			*				*	*			*		*	**		**†		*		*		
Produits laitiers								*						*	**													
Activité physique			*					Côlon / Rectum							**							**	*		*			
Sédentarité																												
Fruits																												
Légumes (non féculents)																												
Fibres alimentaires															**													
Allaitement					*																							

Convaincant | Probable | Suggéré | Non concluant | Non étudié | Suggéré | Probable | Convaincant

Augmentation du risque — Diminution du risque

* signifie que le niveau de preuve est nouvellement étudié depuis le rapport WCRF/AICR 2007 ou les CUP WCRF/AICR 2010, 2011, 2012, 2013, 2014
** signifie que le niveau de preuve a été modifié depuis le rapport WCRF/AICR 2007 ou les CUP WCRF/AICR 2010, 2011, 2012, 2013, 2014
† consommation de compléments alimentaires à base bêtacarotène à fortes doses, en particulier chez les fumeurs et les personnes exposées à l'amiante

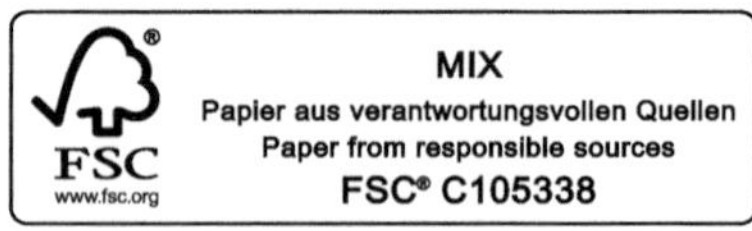

Printed by Books on Demand GmbH, Norderstedt / Germany